MW00990782

This guide is made possible by the support of

Genentech BioOncology™.

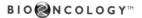

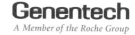

Difficult Conversations

Nurses Share Lessons *from* **Cancer's Frontline**

Difficult Conversations

Nurses Share Lessons *from* Cancer's Frontline

curemediagroup

Dallas, Texas

Published by
CURE Media Group
3102 Oak Lawn, Suite 610
Dallas, Texas 75219
www.curetoday.com

Information presented is not intended as a substitute for the personalized professional advice given by a healthcare provider. The publishers urge readers to contact appropriately qualified health professionals for advice on any health or lifestyle change inspired by information herein.

This publication was produced by CURE Media Group through the financial support of Genentech BioOncology™. The views expressed in this publication are not necessarily those of Genentech BioOncology™ or the publishers. Although great care has been taken to ensure accuracy, CURE Media Group and its servants or agents shall not be responsible or in any way liable for the continued currency of the information or for any errors, omissions or inaccuracies in this book, whether arising from negligence or otherwise or for any consequences arising there from. Review and creation of content is solely the responsibility of CURE Media Group.

Any mention of retail products does not constitute an endorsement by the authors or the publisher.

Library of Congress Control Number: 2011939367

ISBN 978-0-980130867

Written by Kathy LaTour
Medical review provided by Ashley Cothran, RN, OCN; Catherine Cowan, MSN, RN, GNP-BC, AOCNP, CNS-A, WOCN; Renee Genther, ARNP-BC, AOCNP; Deb Harrison, MSN, RN; Annette Jones, BSN, RN, OCN; Sandy Smith, MSN, RN, AOCN; Cynthia Taniguchi, BSN, RN, OCN; Debra Vernon, RN; and Nancy Wells, BSN, RN, OCN

Designed by Susan Douglass
Layout by Glenn Zamora
Photography by Jenny Busing, Richard DeWitt, Matt Rainey, Rob Snavely and Renee Stewart

Printed in the United States of America

Table *of* Contents

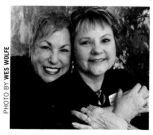

Becky Goodman, BSN,
RN, OCN, [right] with
Kathy LaTour

The Gift of Experience

When I look back on my treatment for breast cancer 25 years ago, I can still hear the voice that calmed my fears during treatment, my oncology nurse Becky Goodman, BSN, RN, OCN. Since then, while traveling the cancer journey with many friends and family, I have seen numerous oncology nurses like Becky in action, and I marvel at their shared talents of compassion and competence. Knowing these skills are not taught in a classroom, I have often wondered where they learned the wisdom of healers. Now I know their insights come from being present for their patients—at the bedside, in the infusion room, on the telephone—and from their colleagues, seasoned nurses who pass their gifts of experience to future generations of nurses.

In the pages that follow, we have captured those conversations: they guide patients through the maze of feelings that come with a cancer diagnosis. They are difficult conversations but essential, and offer to nurses new to these roles—or those who seek them in the future—a glimpse of the best of their profession.

As oncology nurses take on the added roles of nurse specialist, nurse navigator and nurse practitioner, they are now more directly linked to the care of cancer patients than ever before. Far from the classroom, the lessons in this book take you to the heart of the nursing experience: Telling a patient he or she has cancer. Confirming that an advance directive is followed. Ensuring patients take their oral medication. Being present at the end of life.

In these conversations you will find more than 200 years of combined experience from seven nurses who have added special skills to their nursing portfolio.

These moments are real, as are the nurses who share them. They are offered to you as the gift of experience.

Kathy LaTour
CURE's **Editor-at-Large**

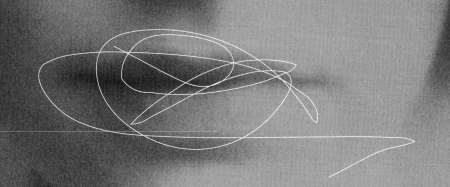

[*Chapter 1*]

A Hard Conversation

[Chapter 1]

A Hard Conversation

Cindi Cantril, MPH, RN, OCN, recalls when she began her career in the early '70s that nurses were not allowed to tell patients their blood pressure. Today, Cantril spends her days with patients who are undergoing breast biopsies—patients who may have cancer. They are conversations that Cantril has prepared for through years of study and nursing.

"Nurses have the time to hold, both literally and figuratively, their patients while they cope with the news," Cantril says. As a program manager for cancer support services and patient navigation, Cantril draws on almost 40 years of experience to find the most supportive way to say, "I am sorry. The biopsy results came back showing cancer cells." She says, "I have an hour or two hours or whatever it takes to hold the patient during the process."

SETTING THE STAGE

Studies show that the stress of waiting for biopsy results can be more intense than the procedure to treat the disease. "It's that kind of anxiety and an existential time for them," she says. "They think they are going to die."

Because Cantril sees patients prior to biopsy, she not only gathers preliminary information but also evaluates their ability to cope with a potential cancer diagnosis. Cantril begins by observing patients' body language and assessing their emotional states, which she calls "setting the stage."

It starts with finding the best time to tell a woman her biopsy result is positive for cancer. "I think the best communication flow is to have patients physically come back

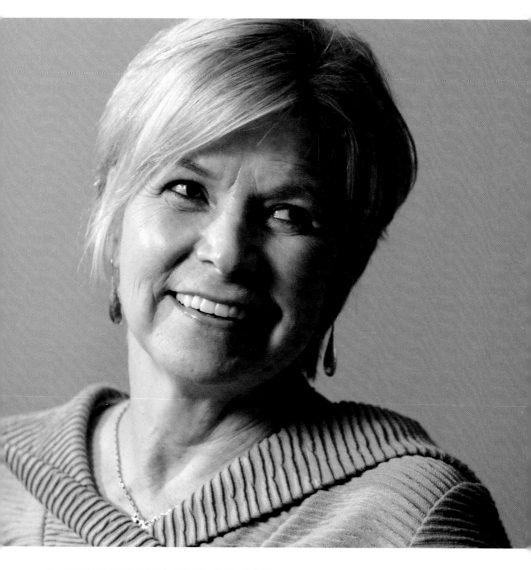

CINDI CANTRIL, MPH, RN, OCN, is a program manager for cancer support services and patient navigation at Sutter Pacific Medical Foundation in Santa Rosa, California. She has served in multiple roles in oncology since the beginning of her professional career. She has taught nurses in a number of settings and was founding vice president of the Oncology Nursing Society in 1975.

for their biopsy results. If your pathology department is going to take three days, ten days, or whatever amount of time, the ideal, particularly for those patients who you believe are going to be positive for cancer, is to physically have them come in."

Before patients arrive for their follow-up appointment, Cantril has called their primary care doctor and made an appointment with the surgeon or medical oncologist.

"The trap I've gotten into in the past is when you don't have a physical appointment with a patient and you call them and say, 'I've got your biopsy results back.' Of course they're going to say, 'Why don't you just tell me what they are?'"

Cantril says that one breast center she knows about tells all patients they will return three days after their biopsy. If their biopsy results are benign, as is the case in about 80 percent of patients, those patients are called with the results and told they don't need to come in for their appointment.

"I am totally mindful that my words will forever change their life."

Cantril shudders at past procedures where patients were told over the phone that they had cancer, even though they might have been driving on the highway with children in the car or at work or listening to voicemail messages. Today, if they cannot come into the office, she asks when is a good time to call back, so they will be home and can talk. Patients have told her they were glad they were home and not at the office because they wanted to be with their spouses, kids or pets.

She says, "I am totally mindful that my words will forever change their life."

STARTING THE JOURNEY

No matter where a patient is in the biopsy process, Cantril says it's important to validate their fears. "I tell patients that I am their GPS. No matter where they are in the system, I know where they are and what's happening. I give them my cell number,

TIPS/TOOLBOX

DISCUSSION STRATEGIES

1 **Find a mentor**—one who can model for you the delivery of difficult news. Be with them to learn and listen.

2 **Develop and trust your own style.** Ask a colleague to observe you and give feedback afterward.

3 **Document your conversations.**

4 **Assess your institutional support** and ask for it repeatedly if you must.

5 **Work within a team.** Remember you are a part of one.

6 **Take care of yourself** like you do others.

RESOURCES

The Oncology Nursing Society has published *Psychosocial Dimensions of Oncology Nursing Care,* which discusses nurse-patient communication. You can find the book and other ONS communication resources at **ons.org**.

The Joint Commission has resources for patient-provider communications at **jointcommission.org**.

The *Journal of Clinical Nursing* published "Nurse-Patient Communication: An Exploration of Patients' Experiences," a study found at **ncbi.nlm.nih.gov/pubmed/14687292**.

The journal *Cancer Nursing* explores the discussion process in "Nurse-Patient Communication in Cancer Care: A Review of the Literature," which can be found at **journals.lww.com/cancernursingonline/ Abstract/2000/02000/Nurse_Patient_ Communication_in_Cancer_Care__A.4.aspx**.

Patient Education and Counseling published "Patient–Health Care Provider Communication During Chemotherapy Treatment: The Perspectives of Women with Breast Cancer," a study that can be found at **sciencedirect.com/science/article/pii/ S0738399100001476**.

CURE ARTICLES

"Layman's Terms" BY CHARLOTTE HUFF, 2009
curetoday.com/index.cfm/fuseaction/article.show/id/2/article_id/1307

"Diagnosis Disclosure" BY TERESA McUSIC, 2011
curetoday.com/index.cfm/fuseaction/journey.show Article/id/9/
enableStageSubMenu/1/article_id/1674

"Making the Most of a Portal" BY MARC SILVER, 2007
curetoday.com/index.cfm/fuseaction/article.show/id/2/article_id/293

"What Really Helps" BY LORI HOPE, 2007
curetoday.com/index.cfm/fuseaction/article.show/id/2/article_id/220

and it's never been abused. Often when I call a patient I am concerned about, he or she will say, 'I cannot believe you are calling me from home.' My reply is that 'It is five minutes out of my life that may forever affect yours.'"

Cantril urges nurses to validate and witness what is happening to the patient; then, gently move him or her forward in developing a plan. As she works to create an optimal environment for having this difficult conversation, Cantril tries to engage all the senses.

"The visual component is particularly important," she says. "When I tell patients their results, I sit down with them and go over every word in their pathology report."

She engages patients through pictures and models of the breast and asks if they want to see the mammography images, because she knows a diagnosis can feel very abstract to them since they may have no physical symptoms. "I can't tell you how many hundreds and hundreds of women have said to me, 'I can't have breast cancer. I don't feel anything. I feel fine. I have no symptoms.' Taking them in and showing them the area on their [scans] makes it more real to them."

Cantril assesses whether the patient can hear what is being said and recommends he or she take a voice recorder to their surgeon's office. "I give them a copy of their pathology report, and I help them formulate questions to ask their doctor. So it's about the physical, emotional, auditory and all the things that we know about how people learn best."

She tells patients that this is an emotional emergency but not a physical emergency. Even with more advanced cancer, she tells them it is not life threatening at the moment, but rather life challenging. "It's tough," Cantril says. "I am a seasoned oncology nurse, and I realize on Fridays that I have rocked people's world all week long."

Cantril says she lets the conversation ebb and flow with tissues and tea. She employs a technique taught to her by a firefighter who found that when people are shaking, they are calmed by the act of holding a cup because they focus on how the cup feels.

"If you can, try to get the patient to focus. Sometimes I tell patients to take a deep breath in through the nose, blow it out slowly through the mouth, and try to just listen as I go through it, and I will write it all down step by step."

MAKING A PLAN

Cantril then describes who the patient will see and in what order. In one instance, she went through all the details with a patient who then told her she had canceled an upcoming vacation.

"I spent two hours with her around all the planning, but I said, 'Call your husband right now and see if he can recapture that trip.'" Cantril then rescheduled all the woman's appointments to allow her to leave on vacation and know what the plan would be when she came back.

"Once patients have a plan, that's what they need. They need somebody to sit down and give them a plan. The worst thing that can happen to patients, in my opinion, is getting a call from the doctor to call them back. When they do, the office is closed, and then the primary care doctor finally gets hold of them and tells them their diagnosis. And then they say, 'What do I do now?' 'Now you have to call the surgeon's office.' Patients are often in complete shock."

The answer to this is patient navigation, Cantril says, and the woman and her vacation is a perfect example. "I set all the things that she needed to do and yet made sure that she had the ability to go on vacation. It wasn't that the medical system was so rigid. It was that she didn't know that she had the right to ask. She didn't know that she could figure that out.

"This person comes to you with a life, and we can try to not let it control his or her life at the very beginning since we know it is going to take over very quickly."

Cantril also concedes that there are some nurses who don't want to give bad news, which she understands.

"I think they have to know their own limitations and know what they feel comfortable doing and not doing, and there is no shame in that."

Cantril says nurses are taught to manage their emotions in nursing school. "My emotions are very clear because I have a delicate balance of what I hope is a sensitive, loving, caring, compassionate demeanor with patients. But I am also strong because they need to hold onto that strength." ⌒

Sexuality and Fertility

Sexuality and Fertility

Beth Schurr, RN, OCN, began her nursing career at age 21 working in cardiology, where she often discussed sexuality with patients as part of their discharge. Schurr says she became aware of the importance of bringing up the subject of sexuality when she asked a male patient whether he had any questions about sexuality and his cardiac disease.

"He said, 'You're the first person who's asked me that. As a matter of fact, I do have a lot of sexual issues as a result of [a medication] that I'm taking, and I've never asked anyone.'" Schurr referred him to a nurse practitioner to discuss side effects. A few days later when she saw the patient again, he thanked her, and added that he never would have told anyone had she not asked.

"I think it totally changed my whole view on why it's important for us to discuss sex with patients," says Schurr, whose experience with cardiology patients carries over to the patients she now treats as an inpatient hematology nurse in the malignant hematology unit at the H. Lee Moffitt Cancer Center. Schurr encourages nurses to simply start the conversation and leave the rest to the patient.

TALKING ABOUT SEX

Schurr doesn't consider herself an expert on sexuality, but her interest has grown over time. Today, she is involved in efforts to add sexual issues to admission and discharge forms for oncology patients.

"We feel comfortable talking with people about their last bowel movement, how to take care of very complex wounds and how to take medications," she says. "But a

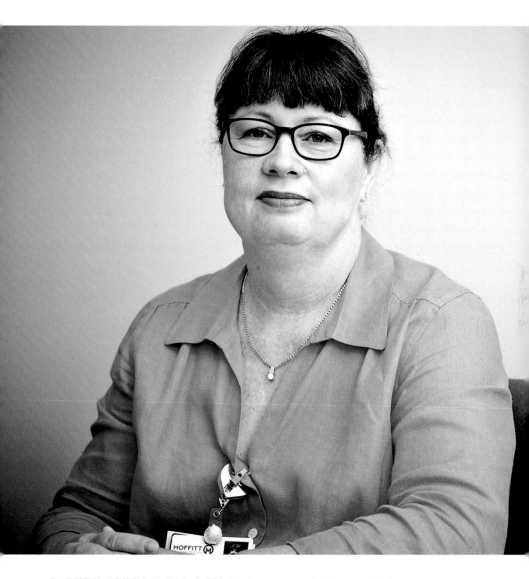

BETH SCHURR, RN, OCN, *has been a nurse for 31 years. For the past five years, she has specialized in oncology as an inpatient hematology nurse at the H. Lee Moffitt Cancer Center in Tampa, Florida, where she teaches nurses about sexuality and cancer.*

fundamental part of people's lives is sex, and it is too often not addressed."

She concedes that the subject is more frequently addressed when the cancer is seen to be connected to sexuality, such as breast, prostate and gynecological cancers. But too often in the general oncology population, it's just not addressed unless a patient brings it up. "And we all know that patients infrequently bring it up," Schurr says.

Schurr reminds the nurses she educates that it doesn't take much to bring up the topic. "It's not like you have to ask a whole lot of probing questions. Sometimes I just say, 'Are you interested in finding out when you can resume sexual activity?'"

The responses will vary, she says, with some saying they aren't worried or there isn't a problem. In those cases, Schurr affirms their decision and tells them that they can discuss sexual issues later, if needed. Others will say they don't need to talk now but want to know who to call when they do need advice. "But a lot of patients say, 'Wow, I'm glad you said that because I was worried about it, and I wasn't going to say anything.'"

Schurr reminds nurses that their job is not to know all the answers but to open the door. "I don't have a PhD in sex, just like I'm not an expert on pain," she says. "We have people whose area of expertise is pain. So, if we have an issue with pain, we bring those people in."

Schurr says, with a laugh, that the biggest hurdle in getting nurses to discuss sexuality is getting them to think about discussing sexuality amid all their other responsibilities. "They forget," Schurr says, "that sexuality is an important part of their patients' lives."

Sexual issues arise from both the physical and emotional aspects of cancer. Schurr has seen the specific sexual issues that affect hematology patients firsthand.

"One of the biggest issues is a result of the effect of the chemotherapy and disease on their bone marrow," she says. "They don't fight off infection well, and they don't make platelets, which prevent bleeding. So for them, sexual activity may not be possible until their counts recover because of the risk of bleeding or the risk of infection."

Schurr brings it up with patients by reminding them that they can generally resume most sexual activity when their platelet count reaches 50,000 and adds that they need to use adequate lubrication to prevent irritating or tearing skin that could result in bleeding.

TIPS/TOOLBOX

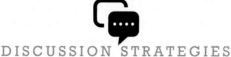

DISCUSSION STRATEGIES

1 **Don't be afraid to introduce the subject of sexuality.** It doesn't have to be a long conversation but can open the door to future conversations.

2 **A meaningful conversation can be prompted by a meaningful question,** such as, "Are you interested in finding out about sexual activity and your disease?"

3 **Nurses open the door** for other professionals to step through.

RESOURCES

The American Cancer Society has information on fertility at **cancer.org/Treatment/TreatmentsandSideEffects/PhysicalSideEffects/FertilityandCancerWhatAreMyOptions/index**. It also has sexuality information for women at **cancer.org/Treatment/TreatmentsandSideEffects/PhysicalSideEffects/SexualSideEffectsinWomen/SexualityfortheWoman/sexuality-for-the-woman-with-cancer-toc** and for men at **cancer.org/Treatment/TreatmentsandSideEffects/PhysicalSideEffects/SexualSideEffectsinMen/SexualityfortheMan/sexuality-for-the-man-with-cancer-toc**.

Find tools and patient education materials on fertility at **fertilehope.org, Myoncofertility.org** and **savemyfertility.org**.

To read more on sexuality, visit the National Cancer Institute website at **cancer.gov/cancertopics/pdq/supportivecare/sexuality/HealthProfessional/page1**.

CURE ARTICLES

"What to Expect When You're Not Expecting—Yet" BY ERIK NESS, 2010
curetoday.com/index.cfm/fuseaction/article.show/id/2/article_id/1482

"Disjointed Custody" BY CHARLOTTE HUFF, 2009
curetoday.com/index.cfm/fuseaction/article.show/id/2/article_id/1154

"Fertility and Family" SIDEBAR IN SUPPLEMENT, 2009
curetoday.com/index.cfm/fuseaction/article.show/id/2/article_id/1295

"At Diagnosis: Special Issues by Age" RESOURCE GUIDE, 2011
curetoday.com/index.cfm/fuseaction/article.show/id/2/article_id/1011

"Sex and Intimacy After Cancer" BY LACEY MEYER, 2010
curetoday.com/index.cfm/fuseaction/article.show/id/2/article_id/1484

"Under the Sheets" BY ELIZABETH WHITTINGTON, 2009
curetoday.com/index.cfm/fuseaction/article.showArticleByTumorType/id/805/tumorCategory/Breast/article_id/1300

"Finding Sensuality After Cancer" BY KATHY LaTOUR, 2010
curetoday.com/index.cfm/fuseaction/article.showArticleByTumorType/id/805/tumorCategory/Breast/article_id/1599

DISCUSSING FERTILITY

Discussions about fertility, a significant problem for many younger hematology patients, are sometimes more challenging than talking about sex, Schurr says.

She recalls having a discussion with a 27-year-old woman about her treatment plan and that it would likely cause infertility. When Schurr began talking with her, the young woman said she was feeling overwhelmed and needed the information in smaller doses. The first conversation, Schurr recalls, was telling the patient she would be given a medication to stop her period to keep her from bleeding excessively when her counts went down. Schurr says, "She found out she had a life-threatening disease, and then, in addition, she learned she probably won't be able to have children."

Unlike many cancers where patients have time to address sperm banking or egg retrieval, Schurr says that with acute leukemia, patients usually have to be treated

Some patients have a diminished sense of touch or smell due to chemotherapy treatments, and senses are important to the sexual experience.

immediately, which makes those efforts nearly impossible. If they have time to address fertility, Schurr says, ideally those services would be available at their cancer center, and if not, at least they could be provided a referral source so that patients don't have to seek out specialists on their own, as is commonly the case now.

Schurr says it was a fertility discussion that led to a humorous moment with a 19-year-old patient. After his doctors told him about the probable loss of fertility, he told Schurr and his mother that he didn't want to be treated. "We were both shocked. I said rather bluntly, 'Would you rather be infertile or dead? That's your option here,'" Schurr says.

The confused look on the young man's face prompted Schurr to ask him what he thought infertile meant. He said it meant he would never have sex again. After Schurr explained that infertility didn't mean he would be impotent but that he may be sterile, he responded that he would go ahead with treatment. Schurr says she couldn't resist asking him whether he would still go through treatment even if it meant he couldn't have sex again, and he said he would have to think about it.

RECOGNIZING HEALING

With the population of survivors growing, Schurr says it is becoming more important to discuss sexuality as treatment ends. Almost 70 percent of breast cancer survivors report having sexual issues, and the same goes for about 80 percent of prostate cancer patients.

"Starting to talk about sexuality in different kinds of cancer populations is a big discussion," she says. "For example, gastrointestinal cancer patients who have colostomies. That can put a real damper on a sex life, not to mention the changes to body image."

Some patients have a diminished sense of touch or smell due to chemotherapy treatments, and senses are important to the sexual experience, Schurr adds.

In addition to sexual performance and body image, an issue some patients deal with is role reversal as their partner becomes the caregiver or becomes responsible for providing all the financial support for the family. "Sexuality is not just the act of having sex; it's all the things that go along with it," Schurr says. "It's such a complex thing."

Cancer's impact on sexuality remains under-researched, Schurr says, adding that she can find volumes of studies on preventing constipation but very little on practical interventions for sexual issues. Cancer patients deal with issues such as decreased libido, changes in body function, surgical late effects and overall body image.

Nurses make sure their patients have their pain medication and know when their next appointment is, Schurr says. "We provide counseling for financial issues and childcare and all these things, but we don't think about addressing sexuality with patients."

Many nurses say they feel more comfortable talking to patients about the end of their life and hospice care, Schurr says. "And yet sexuality doesn't get brought up."

"We can deal with death better than we can with sex," she adds. "I think that's a very interesting commentary on our society as a whole." ∾

[*Chapter 3*]

Oral Therapy
Adherence

[*Chapter 3*]

Oral Therapy Adherence

Jody Pelusi, PhD, FNP, AOCNP, recalls a young patient well: a single mother with breast cancer, who couldn't work, had struggled through her intravenous adjuvant chemotherapy and was elated when it ended. She was ready to "get back to normal," says Pelusi, a 38-year oncology nurse.

Pelusi had prepared the woman for more treatment—a pill she would need to take every day for the next five years. She says the patient understood the pill was part of her treatment and the goal of treatment was curative. What the patient didn't realize was that the medicine had side effects because she assumed most pills don't have them.

"When some of the menopausal-type side effects from her hormonal therapy started occurring, her way of dealing with it was to stop taking her pill as prescribed," Pelusi says. "She didn't want to mention the side effects to me because she didn't want to be seen as always complaining. In her mind, she just wanted to feel better again and get on with her life." The patient didn't comprehend that routinely missing doses could adversely affect the outcome of her treatment. Pelusi sensed she was struggling. It took Pelusi several months of trying multiple strategies and providing considerable education as she tackled one symptom after another. During this time, she approached the patient as a partner with carefully chosen language that was not accusatory.

"I put the words on me," Pelusi says. "I asked, 'What can I do to help you? If you explain the symptoms you are having, we can figure out together what to do to make them better.'"

Pelusi had the patient keep a journal of what she ate, how she felt and what she was doing when hot flashes occurred. With this, Pelusi was able to identify that a glass of

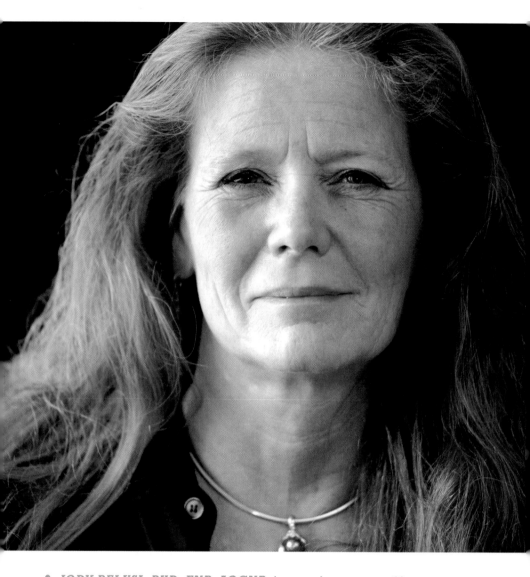

JODY PELUSI, PHD, FNP, AOCNP, is an oncology nurse practitioner and researcher at Arizona Oncology in Sedona. She is active at the national, state and local levels and has had four-year appointments to the FDA Oncological Drug Advisory Committee, FDA Oncology Pediatric Subcommittee and FDA Quality of Life Subcommittee. She previously served on the Oncology Nursing Society's Board of Directors.

wine, caffeine and increased stress might be spurring her hot flashes. She also assisted the patient in creating an exercise, nutrition and stress-management plan and checked on her routinely to ensure she was motivated to take the medication as prescribed.

"Every patient is different," Pelusi says. "We have to know how putting this pill in their lives will affect them. These are not five-minute conversations."

Finally, Pelusi was able to reduce the patient's symptoms without stopping or adding medication. "People start on oral cancer therapies, and their perception is that they should have few, if any, side effects," Pelusi says. "It's our responsibility as physicians, nurse practitioners and nurses to ensure patients have as few side effects as possible or none at all."

A GROWING PROBLEM

The challenges around oral cancer therapy adherence are well known in the oncology community and to Pelusi, who chaired the Oral Cancer Therapy Task Force for US Oncology (now McKesson Specialty Health) in 2011. She is among many who focus on identifying and addressing issues of adherence as oral chemotherapy drugs become more prevalent—estimates are that 25 percent of cancer therapies will be administered orally by 2013.

Currently, non-adherence rates for oral chemotherapy drugs range from 30 to 50 percent. Non-adherence is a major concern since it ultimately affects the patient's response to treatment and the overall outcome. Patients stop or cut down on their medication for a number of reasons, including unmanaged side effects, not understanding the goal of therapy, confusion about when and how to take the medication, complexity of dosing schedules, motivation and duration of taking the medication, and cost.

Cost has become a significant barrier. According to a study presented at the 2011 American Society of Clinical Oncology annual meeting, up to 10 percent of patients never fill their first oral cancer therapy prescription because of out-of-pocket costs or the complexity of taking the drug.

"Until someone starts an oral medication, we don't know how it will affect them," Pelusi says. "In addition, most patients are on other medications, which can contribute

TIPS/TOOLBOX

DISCUSSION STRATEGIES

1 **Remember to** present information as "we are in this together."

2 **Educate patients** about the medication at a second appointment after they have had time to fully understand the diagnosis.

3 **Thoroughly instruct** the patient about the medication's side effects and interactions and have the patient sign a consent form agreeing to take the medication according to instructions.

4 **Use a symptom tracker.**

5 **Use a "teach back" method** with patients. Ask them to repeat what you have said.

6 **Ask patients to be honest** about side effects and work to eliminate them.

7 **Discuss safety** issues in handling the drugs.

8 **Use special calendars** and pill bottles to avoid confusion.

RESOURCES

Many pharmaceutical companies provide support for patients and nurses with toll-free numbers and websites. Check the drug's manufacturer for patient assistance programs and nurse support.

Healthcare professionals can customize treatment plans at **medactionplan.com** and share them on **mymedschedule.com** with patients and families.

Coach 4 Cancer provides worksheets to give to patients at **coach4cancer.com/charts.pdf**.

The Oncology Nursing Society (ONS) has a tool kit for addressing patient concerns and problems about oral chemotherapy adherence at **ons.org/ClinicalResources/OralTherapies/media/ons/ docs/clinical/AdherenceToolkit/toolkit.pdf**.

CURE ARTICLES

"Use as Directed" BY LAURA BEIL, 2007
curetoday.com/index.cfm/fuseaction/article.show/id/2/article_id/204

"Q&A: Taking Meds as Prescribed" BY LEN LICHTENFELD, MD, 2010
curetoday.com/index.cfm/fuseaction/article.show/id/2/article_id/1536

A Patient's Guide to Medication Adherence 2007
media.curetoday.com/downloads/documents/pocketguide_adherence_forweb.pdf

to side effects."

When the patient's oral chemotherapy prescription is filled, Pelusi asks them to bring in all the medications and supplements that they are taking, so she can review what interactions may occur as the new medication is being introduced. She also wants to ensure they can negotiate drug packaging. Illustrating this point, Pelusi recalls an instance where a patient with arthritis was unable to easily open a blister pack. In cases such as this, alternative packaging would need to be requested from the pharmacy provider.

Packaging of medication may also be an issue with pill bottles. "If [the pharmacy] puts it all in one bottle, we take out one week to be sure they don't get confused. It sounds like a lot of work, but you get into a routine after doing it time and time again."

When citing an example of a drug interaction, she recalls a patient who fell and broke his collarbone while on a camping trip. At the hospital, he began having heart issues.

Perhaps the greatest challenge in addressing adherence is that there is no one-size-fits-all solution for educating patients.

When his healthcare team contacted Pelusi, she advised discontinuing his oral chemotherapy until his heart problems cleared up. He continued to experience complications. When Pelusi saw him a few months later, she said "Let's get you back on your oral treatment." The patient told her he never stopped taking the chemotherapy; his wife sneaked it to him every day. "He kept having these complications [because his chemotherapy was] interfering with some of those drugs he was being given at the hospital."

Pelusi recounts another situation. "I have a patient who is 84, and she tells me her oral drugs have made her bowling better, but it's because she feels better. She knows she will not be cured. She knows the medicine is keeping her cancer in check. She can go bowling and be with her daughter." When the patient experienced side effects, Pelusi suggested lowering the dose, but the patient disagreed.

"I told her I wanted her to be in the bowling tournament but if the side effects got worse she would not be able to participate. I said, 'Let's go down by one pill now, and we'll get a scan in a few months. If it's good, then we'll know that it is still working. If it's not, then we'll go back on the medication.' We know from studies that 40 percent of all patients have to have a dose reduction, and they still get the same outcome from the medication. Therefore, it is not unusual to have a dose reduction."

Research shows that routine assessment, ongoing patient education, proactive symptom management and strong nurse-provider-patient relationships contribute to optimal adherence. Pelusi also asserts that having a formalized plan and process for oral cancer therapies in a practice will provide consistency and efficiency in care and, in the process, enhance adherence and patient, family and staff satisfaction.

MEETING CHALLENGES

Perhaps the greatest challenge in addressing adherence is that there is no one-size-fits-all solution for educating patients. Nurses must play multiple roles with each patient. Once treatment options have been reviewed with the patient and oral medication has been decided on, the patient is scheduled for a return visit in a few days.

"These are long conversations. I have a lot of follow-up. Sometimes I feel like a broken record. But every time I go into a room, I tell myself that I hear it 25 times a day, but it's the first time they are hearing it," Pelusi says.

In talking with patients, she maintains a nonjudgmental tone. "Choose your words carefully. Don't say, 'Did you.' Instead say, 'I have had patients in the past who have had a hard time taking their oral medications around the holidays or affording them. Is that something that is familiar to you?'" Pelusi emphasizes the responsibility to patients to take their meds as prescribed. At this point, compliance becomes a matter of regular follow-up—a crucial aspect of adherence that may come not only from the patient's oncology team but also from outside monitoring agency nurses or specialty pharmacies.

Pelusi recalls a story about a patient, a college professor who was worried about her colleagues seeing her take medication. Pelusi thought she had worked through the patient's concerns when she received a call from an oncology nurse with the pharmaceutical company's patient assistance program who was doing phone follow-up. The patient admitted to the pharmaceutical company nurse that she was taking both doses at breakfast, so she wouldn't have to take the second pill at the school.

"She told a nurse on the phone, but not me," Pelusi says. "She was afraid I would take her off the medication if I knew she wasn't taking it correctly but thought the monitoring nurse, whom she had never met, couldn't stop her medication. Monitoring nurses and pharmacists don't replace what we do but rather reinforce what we've said and done," Pelusi explains. "They are our extra set of eyes and ears to help us know what the patient is doing in terms of dosing and what side effects the patient may be experiencing." Pelusi called the patient and advised that if the drug was putting this much stress in her life, it might not be the drug for her.

> ## "We must place ourselves in our patients' shoes and try to understand how these medications fit into their daily lives."

"We need to create an environment with many safety checks, a lot of support and education and ongoing evaluation of their experiences and outcomes," Pelusi says. "We must place ourselves in our patients' shoes and try to understand how these medications fit into their daily lives, so we can have the skills and insight to properly care for them. It takes a team and, many times, that team includes outside pharmacists and nurses."

Pelusi discusses medication safety with her patients and the practical aspects of taking a drug that could be harmful if swallowed by a child or pet. "It is all about safety, communication and commitment. It's about restructuring our practices, and it won't take a lot," she says.

"Oral cancer therapies are our future, and the time is now to make sure we have prepared ourselves and our practices to efficiently and effectively manage them." ⌒

[*Chapter 4*]

Facing Recurrence

[*Chapter 4*]

Facing Recurrence

Brenda Howard, MA, RN, OCN, a nursing education specialist at H. Lee Moffitt Cancer Center in Tampa, Florida, says most patients are in shock when they learn their cancer is back. And high-risk patients live with the fear of recurrence all the time, says Howard.

For those who do receive the news of recurrence, Howard tells nurses not to just stand there but to get eye level: "I get down on their level if I have to get down on my knees and hold their hands or hold them while they cry. We all need touch."

Howard recalls a time when there were few, if any, options for those whose cancer had recurred, "and now there are multiple patients who are on their fifth or sixth different treatment regimen." She asks them to talk about the fears the news of a recurrence brings. "Usually it's that they are afraid of being a burden," she says. "Also, not being able to provide for the family and not having the financial resources." Howard encourages patients to move forward one day at a time, or if that's too much, to only look at the next hour—or even the next five minutes.

Language is important. "We don't talk about dying so much as about living. I think it's important how it's phrased to patients. I can remember, years ago, filling in for another nurse with a breast surgeon. This woman had come in for her yearly mammogram, and they found a new tumor underneath one of her breast implants. He said to her, 'We're going to do salvage therapy.' And she looked at him, and she said, 'Salvage therapy? I am not garbage. I am a human being.' Patients come in extremely vulnerable. And if their cancer has recurred, they're pretty low to begin with. So, we need to watch what we say and how we say it."

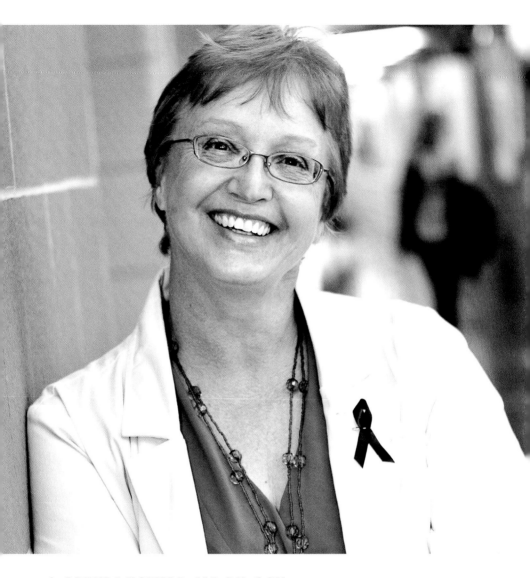

BRENDA HOWARD, MA, RN, OCN, has worked in numerous aspects of oncology since beginning her nursing career in 1975. She has taught many levels of nursing at a number of hospitals and coordinated oncology programs for H. Lee Moffitt Cancer Center since 2008.

Pain might accompany a recurrence, which brings up questions about how much pain to expect and how the pain will be treated. Most large cancer centers have palliative care or pain clinics with specialists who are very good at helping manage intractable pain, she says. For those patients at small centers where such specialties don't exist, she recommends looking at the closest cancer center geographically. As far as integrative therapy is concerned, massage can do wonders for decreasing pain and anxiety in cancer patients, when it's appropriate.

Everyone is afraid of the unknown, Howard says. While working in a surgical gynecological practice, she saw this fear in patients with a high risk of ovarian cancer recurrence who called her to check their blood work before their follow-up appointments. The fear of recurrence was so powerful, sometimes patients were positive the cancer was back when it wasn't. "You look at all of the hard facts: the scans, the lab work, and then if they're okay, you have to sit down face to face," she says.

Howard says it's not a phone conversation, but one during which she sits with the patient to discuss what is going on in the patient's life and to address the anxiety that brings on this fear. "It takes time," she adds, "but it really establishes a bond between me and that patient. And then the patient trusts me. So if something does go wrong, I've already established that trust."

Howard recalls a patient named Jane, who had been treated for ovarian cancer. She called Howard complaining of aches in her joints, sure that the cancer had recurred in her bones. Her stomach was acting up, and she was stressed out.

"Her blood work didn't show anything, and her scans were clean. I sat down and said, 'Okay, Jane, tell me, what's going on in your life? What's happening to you outside of the hospital?' We sat and talked about problems she was having in the family and how she was coping with her family—which she wasn't; she wasn't coping with them at all. We were able to get our social worker in to work with her and the family. And that helped ease some of that tension."

ECONOMIC REALITY

Perhaps the most pressing issue for patients facing treatment a second time is cost.

TIPS/TOOLBOX

DISCUSSION STRATEGIES

1 Be there. Don't have difficult conversations over the phone. Get on the patient's level and look them in the eyes. Hold the patient's hand. Hold them if they cry.

2 Understand. The fear of recurrence is a powerful force, and those who think their cancer has returned may be responding to outside factors.

3 Help patients to know that they will not be abandoned even if there are no further treatment options.

4 Learn about cancer economics and the cost of additional treatment.

5 Know that the greatest fear is fear of the unknown.

RESOURCES

The American Cancer Society has information on understanding recurrence at **cancer.org/Treatment/SurvivorshipDuringandAfterTreatment/ UnderstandingRecurrence/index**.

Learn more about coping with a recurrence at the Mayo Clinic website at **mayoclinic.com/health/cancer/CA00050**.

Information about cancer recurrence from the American Society for Clinical Oncology is available at **cancer.net/patient/All+About+Cancer/Treating+Cancer/ Dealing+With+Cancer+Recurrence**.

CURE ARTICLES

"The Cancer Chronicles" BY KATHY LaTOUR, 2006
curetoday.com/index.cfm/fuseaction/article.show/id/2/article_id/484

"After Treatment: Fear of Recurrence"
CANCER RESOURCE GUIDE 2011, WEB EXCLUSIVE
curetoday.com/index.cfm/fuseaction/article.show/id/2/article_id/995

"Predicting Recurrence"
CANCER RESOURCE GUIDE 2011, WEB EXCLUSIVE
curetoday.com/index.cfm/fuseaction/article.show/id/2/article_id/1001

"Facing Down the Fear" BY LORI HOPE, 2008
curetoday.com/index.cfm/fuseaction/article.show/id/2/article_id/648

"Challenges in Cancer Survivorship"
BY KATHY LaTOUR, 2008
curetoday.com/index.cfm/fuseaction/article.show/id/2/article_id/127

"What Five Years Really Means"
BY CURTIS PESMAN, 2007
curetoday.com/index.cfm/fuseaction/article.show/id/2/article_id/214

Howard says that nurses often don't think about financial issues as often as they should.

"We had ordered this medication for a patient who was having nausea. And I said, 'This is relatively cheap.' She called me back the next day and said, 'I don't know what your idea of cheap is, but you ordered 30 pills, and my copay for each pill is two dollars. That's a water bill.' That's one thing I really stress with nurses now, especially in chemo classes. Nurses should look at the economics to address it with them upfront. I've had patients go bankrupt. They run up their credit cards to the max and then can't figure out how to pay the bills, pay the mortgage or buy food to eat."

Howard recalls hearing from a man whose wife had melanoma. He called with questions because he wanted to take his wife to another cancer center that he heard had a new treatment option. He told Howard he didn't really have the money but wanted to do everything he could for his wife.

"During our conversation, he told me about their expenses, and it was phenomenal. He said, 'I thought that we would have money for our golden years. Let me tell you, they are not golden. We have just dug ourselves into a hole that we can't get out of.'"

These days it can fall on nurses to help patients navigate financial matters. "I know a social worker who says, 'Everybody wants Cadillac care but at Honda prices.' And it's getting to the point where that's not possible anymore. We used to be able to do that in the '90s, but we can't do that anymore. We have to be better stewards of what we're doing because from a business perspective, we're not being reimbursed, and the patients don't even have the money for their copays. If we can offer them any type of treatment or help, we do it. But if we can't, I think it's really important that they understand that we're not abandoning them. That's the big part of it."

If the patient says he or she cannot afford the recommended treatment, Howard says that this should be part of the discussion with the care team who may be able to recommend options, which may not be first-line therapy but something that would keep the patient going.

For example, she says, "We had one lady who had six or seven courses of chemo and was hitting a wall. So the doctor tried a drug that had just been out there forever. I mean it was one of the old, old drugs. And she responded to it somewhat. It was enough to keep her quality of life decent for a few months. Those few months were what she needed because her grandson was graduating from high school, and she wanted to be around to see that. So, for her, that was a doable option."

Knowing what is on the patient's "bucket list" is significant to caring for the patient as a whole. "I think, as we age, those things become more important to us. For this patient, seeing her grandson graduate was something important. Her quality of life was good enough that she could go do that in a wheelchair," Howard says. "When people know that they're up against a wall, we need to reassure them that we are going to do symptom management; that we are not going to abandon them; that their pain will be kept under control; that we'll take care of the symptoms as much as possible."

NO FURTHER OPTIONS

Sometimes the "cancer is back" conversation is followed by the "treatment isn't working" discussion—an exchange that must focus on what the patient wants. Howard recalls a mother of two young autistic sons. After her initial diagnosis of ovarian cancer, her treatment went well. Then the cancer recurred nine months later, coming back with "a vengeance." The few treatment options remaining didn't work.

"Her biggest concern was how her sons were going to manage," Howard says. "It wasn't about how she was going to die; it was about how her sons were going to live."

Howard and a social worker spent time arranging options with the patient's husband. "We put her into hospice fairly quickly so that we could get her support to help her make the decisions she needed to make for these kids. Her husband was very supportive, but he traveled a lot." Howard and the social worker suggested the husband consider job alternatives so he could manage the children. Howard says nurses are better positioned to have such discussions because doctors seldom have the time, although some are better than others.

"Just because they're not in active treatment doesn't mean you're writing them off. When there are no further drugs we can give for the cancer, there are a lot of things we can do to help make them comfortable and to work through this." ⌒

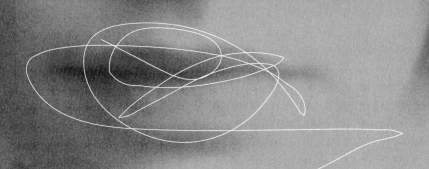

[Chapter 5]

Palliative Care

Palliative Care

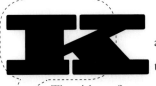athy Plakovic, APRN, AOCNP, AHPCN, begins to tear up when talking about one of the first patients with pain she cared for.

The girl was five years old, had rhabdomyosarcoma in her bones and was screaming in pain.

"They called me in because they hoped to give her some good quality of life for the time she had left," Plakovic recalls. "They were giving her increasing doses of morphine that would help the pain some, but it would sedate her and cause her breathing to slow down. Then they gave her less because they were afraid of killing her."

Plakovic tried two other pain medications, neither of which worked. Finally she started the child on an intravenous medication Plakovic says is used extensively for cancer pain. Since the patient was so young, Plakovic could only estimate the dosage. "It's a long-acting drug once in the system and takes a long time to get out, so if you overshoot your mark, it could be fatal."

The next morning Plakovic walked in to find her young patient sitting up in bed and painting a picture. "It was the most rewarding thing ever to see this little girl able to just be herself."

A PAIN REMEDY

Palliative care focuses on creating the best quality of life for patients who have been diagnosed with a life-limiting or life-threatening illness. This may be through symptom management, such as alleviating pain or nausea with medication. Plakovic says nurses are also often called upon to assist with the psychosocial issues that accompany the

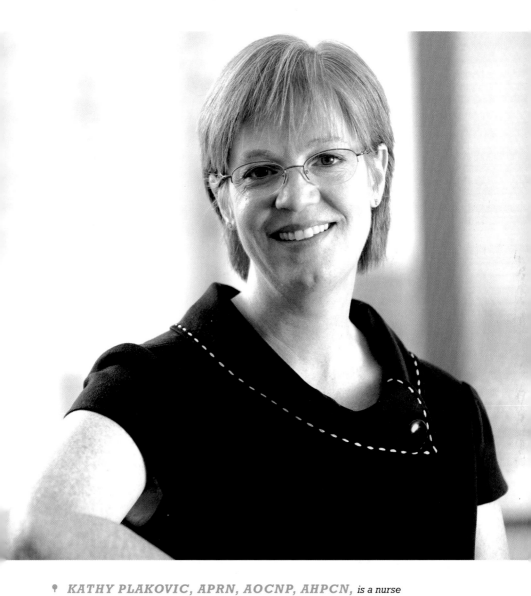

KATHY PLAKOVIC, APRN, AOCNP, AHPCN, *is a nurse practitioner in inpatient palliative care service at* Memorial Sloan-Kettering Cancer Center *in New York. She began her nursing career as a staff nurse in 1989 and started as an oncology nurse in 1993 in Texas, where she also served as the president of the Central Texas Oncology Nursing Society in 2003. She co-authored a chapter on palliative care in* Evidence-Based Ambulatory Care for the Older Adult.

physical issues: depression, hopelessness and anger.

She says, "That's a big part of my job—really having time to sit down with families and talk to them about decisions that need to be made, what they are experiencing and how they can best support their family member."

For many patients, Plakovic says, psychosocial or spiritual issues can have an impact on pain management. She recalls a 35-year-old patient with metastatic rectal cancer who gave birth to her first child the month before her diagnosis.

"She had back pain, some rectal bleeding and constipation during her pregnancy. Everyone said, 'Oh, you're pregnant; that's it.' I met her in urgent care, and she was writhing in pain, awful pain. We were giving her huge doses of medication to try and get it under control."

Palliative care focuses on creating the best quality of life for patients who have been diagnosed with a life-limiting or life-threatening illness.

As Plakovic tried to medicate her, she noticed the patient was distracted by a baby's cries coming from the hall. She learned it was the patient's baby and asked if the baby and its caregiver could go into another area for a while. "She was stressed, and I think hearing her baby cry was not helping her."

After receiving additional medication, the patient was relieved. "I think part of it was that she could hear her child cry and couldn't do anything about it because she was in so much pain herself," Plakovic says. "When you take care of some of the psychological distress that someone's having, you're able to take care of their pain as well. If you're not taking care of the psychological or the spiritual side of things, you're never going to get that pain under control."

Plakovic suspects many younger cancer patients struggle with psychological and spiritual issues because they're coming to terms with their own mortality for the first time.

TIPS/TOOLBOX

DISCUSSION STRATEGIES

1 Listen. Far too many times people want to fill that gap of silence. Just listen—even listen to the silence—and get something more from the patient or family.

2 Educate. Many patients and families are concerned about addiction. Explain that it's unlikely someone will develop an addiction if he or she hasn't previously had one. Tell them that as long as there is pain, a person will not get addicted to these medications.

3 Advocate. Be a tireless advocate for your patients. Don't take no for an answer. If resources, such as social work and psychiatry, are unavailable at your facility, find out what's available in the community.

4 Mediate. If you cannot resolve conflicting viewpoints among the healthcare team, request a review by your center's ethics committee. A committee can interpret documents or help you come to a conclusion that is in the patient's best interest.

RESOURCES

The Center to Advance Palliative Care has information at two different websites: for nurses at **capc.org** and for patients at **getpalliativecare.org**.

The National Hospice and Palliative Care organization sponsors "Caring Connections," which provides resources and information at **caringinfo.org**.

Among other information, the Hospice and Palliative Nurses Association offers patient and family teaching sheets to download that address specific topics, such as managing anxiety and hospice and palliative care at **hpna.org/DisplayPage.aspx?Title=Patient/Family%20Teaching%20Sheets**.

National Institute of Nursing Research has a brochure on palliative care at **ninr.nih.gov/NR/rdonlyres/01CC45F1-048B-468A-BD9F-3AB727A381D2/0/NINR_PalliativeBrochure_Brochure_12_Layout_Version_508.pdf**.

CURE ARTICLES

"The New Specialty in Cancer Care"
BY JOANNE KENEN, 2008
curetoday.com/index.cfm/fuseaction/article.show/id/2/article_id/163

"Another Deafening Silence"
BY BETTY FARRELL, PhD, RN, 2008
curetoday.com/index.cfm/fuseaction/article.show/id/2/article_id/160

"Q & A: Palliative Care Helpful Along the Journey" BY LEN LICHTENFELD, MD, 2010
curetoday.com/index.cfm/fuseaction/article.show/id/2/article_id/1576

"When the Choice is Not Cure"
BY MARC SILVER, SIDEBAR, 2006
curetoday.com/index.cfm/fuseaction/article.show/id/2/article_id/550

She gives an example of a 42-year-old woman with metastatic pancreatic cancer. Plakovic was called in to help her understand how to talk to her children, who were three and five years old. The woman, surrounded by her spouse and extended family, was in significant pain when Plakovic arrived.

After getting the patient's pain under control, Plakovic recommended some resources to help the couple talk to their children. They told her they wanted to make sure the children were aware she was going to die because it was going to happen soon. But more pressing was the woman's desire to get out of the hospital, so she could spend as much time with her children as possible.

"This was Friday afternoon, and the primary team was saying she would be in the hospital over the weekend, so radiation could start on Monday. I found out that, right then, we were waiting on the radiation oncologist to see her." Plakovic got on the phone

Plakovic says it is essential to find out what is important to the patient.

to see if she could expedite the discharge only to have the resident say he had to call his attending physician. Finally, Plakovic called the patient's physician directly.

She told the doctor that the patient was distressed and wanted to go home to see her children. Finally, Plakovic told the radiation oncologist to come right away or the patient would be discharged. The radiation oncologist came and did the consult so she could be discharged. Plakovic says, "She went home and got to see her children. She received her radiation as an outpatient. The following week she went to the Jersey Shore with her kids and had a family vacation. The week after that, she died."

WHAT'S IMPORTANT

Plakovic says it is essential to find out what is important to the patient. In one case, she says, a patient wanted to die at home. The patient was so close to death the team was afraid she would die in the ambulance. They explained this to the patient, who said she understood but still wanted to go home.

"We expedited the hospice referral, got everything in place," Plakovic says. But when Plakovic arrived to check on the patient the next morning, she learned the woman died during the night. "She never made it home, but she knew she was going home. And I think once you know you're heading towards the goal you want, that's what matters."

Sometimes the patient's goal is to control the end of life, and Plakovic says she has had more than one situation where she recognized the importance of having advance directives, such as a living will and a healthcare proxy.

"We had a 73-year-old man who had been diagnosed with colon cancer, treated and was in remission. The cancer recurred, and he kept having things pop up that needed spot treatments." The patient had diabetes and heart disease in addition to cancer. Then, after a radiation procedure, he developed pneumonia and was placed in the hospital's intensive care unit.

"On rounds, I asked if he needed a palliative care referral, and when I saw him, it was clear he wasn't doing well. But it also came to light that he had a living will that was the most comprehensive living will I have ever seen. It was clear what he wanted, which was not to be on a ventilator. He didn't want artificial nutrition and hydration or dialysis."

The patient's wife thought he would make it out of the ICU again, so she wanted the ICU team to try to do what they could to keep him alive, even if it was against his wishes. "The oncologist would not say the cancer was killing him because it wasn't," Plakovic recalls. "It was all the other conditions along with his age. So no one would tell her it was the end of the line."

Plakovic returned the next week to find the patient still in the ICU and in worse condition: his kidneys had failed, and he was on dialysis; he was being fed through a tube and was on a ventilator. "During rounds I asked the ICU team if anyone had talked to him about his living will in the periods when he was alert. I was not being heard. Then the next week on rounds when they were talking about him, the doctor said that when the nurses go in he is crying. It broke my heart. I lost it. I said, 'He let his wishes be known, and we are not following them.' They said, 'The wife's not ready.' I'm like,

'It's not her decision. It's his decision, and he's made it.' So I kind of went around and around with the ICU team. The oncologist was of no help. I felt like he needed an advocate. And so I called an ethics consult."

Plakovic says the hospital's ethics team examined the patient's living will and reviewed his case and agreed with Plakovic that he had left clear instructions about what he had wanted. "We met with the wife, and the wife was devastated because she never heard from anyone that he was dying. She had no idea that he was this close to death. We talked to her about his living will and that he had left clear instructions for her. And he even said in his living will that, 'If my wife, my healthcare agent, is not able to make these decisions, I will allow my physicians to make the decision for her.'" She was upset because she was coming to terms with the fact that he was dying, and she didn't feel that she could make the decision to remove the ventilator, Plakovic says.

"The thing that's most important to me in my job is to know that I made a difference."

"I told her, 'It's not your decision. It's his decision, and he's already made it for you.' And there was sudden relief that I could visibly see on her face because she realized, 'It's not my decision.'" The next day, with a harpist and chaplain in the room, the family gathered, and the patient was taken off the ventilator. He died within minutes.

"The thing that's most important to me in my job is to know that I made a difference," Plakovic says. "If I come in and see a patient having pain, I write [a prescription] for a pain medication. And if the next day, they report that their pain is better—that's a good day. If a family is distressed and doesn't understand the dying process, I talk to them, tell them what to expect and spend time with them and their loved one. And when they come back the next day, and I see them at ease—just being attentive to their loved one while they're dying and not being scared to touch them or to talk to them— I've done my job." ∞

Advance
Directives

[Chapter 6]

Advance Directives

Gabriela Kaplan, MSN, RN, AOCN, counsels nurses that advance directives are important. But even more important is encouraging communication between patients, families and healthcare professionals to help patients make difficult end-of-life decisions.

Kaplan, an oncology nurse since the mid-1970s, has seen the role of oncology nurses expand to include counseling patients about advance directives. The goal of these written instructions is to give patients a voice about their wishes when they can no longer speak for themselves. "I tell my nursing students to look at advance directives and to complete one [for themselves], so they better understand them," Kaplan says.

Although advance directives can take many forms and laws about them vary in each state, the most common documents are directives to physicians, family members and caregivers (sometimes called living wills) that contain a patient's wishes about types of treatment and life-sustaining measures. Another standard document is a medical power of attorney or healthcare proxy, which designates who will make healthcare decisions if the patient becomes incapacitated. In many states, the healthcare proxy has, in essence, the same right to request or refuse treatment that the individual would have.

Kaplan favors a document developed by Aging with Dignity, a nonprofit agency, called "Five Wishes," which combines a living will and medical power of attorney, and addresses comfort care and spirituality. Five Wishes is legally accepted in all but eight states: Alabama, Indiana, Kansas, New Hampshire, Ohio, Oregon, Texas and Utah.

"It's a document or a conversation that you have with someone you love about what you would like in case things don't go well," Kaplan says, adding that when she asks

---

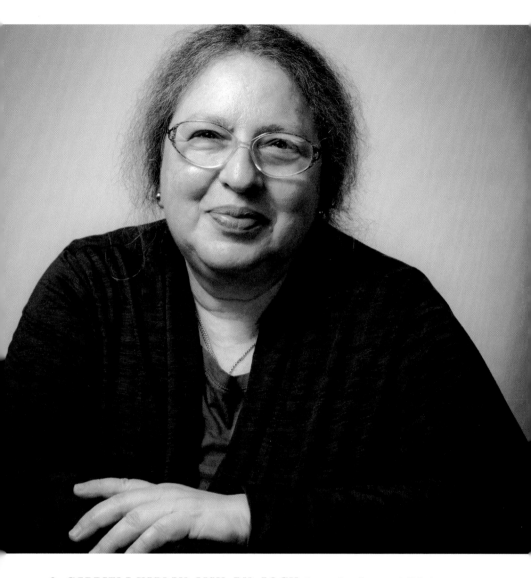

GABRIELA KAPLAN, MSN, RN, AOCN, is an education specialist at
Newark Beth Israel Medical Center in Newark, New Jersey. She began her nursing
career in 1975 and is currently an adjunct faculty member at Trinitas School of
Nursing in Elizabeth, New Jersey. Her research includes ethics, moral distress
and hospice.

patients about care decisions, they will say they have discussed it with family, to which she replies, "Did you put it in writing?"

SO MUCH MORE

Kaplan cautions that hospitals are now required to ask about advance directives and provide information to patients who don't have them. What begins as a piece of paper in a patient's file may take on new complexities when the time comes to apply its meaning. And it's frequently the nurses, Kaplan says, who become arbiters of these discussions.

She recalls an incident early in her career, before the written form of advance directives was common, that involved a patient who had a do not resuscitate (DNR) order. The family knew he was near death, and it had been documented that the physician had told them the patient had requested a DNR.

"I was doing an assessment later that day, and the patient was not looking very good. His respiratory rate was down, and he was getting cold," Kaplan says. At that time, she turned to the man's family and said, "'You know he's really not doing well. This could be it.' His wife looked at me and said, 'Well, do something.' So, I looked at her, and this was one of the hardest sentences I ever said: 'Do you really want me to do something?' And she said, 'Yes.'" Kaplan says she notified the doctors who came in and talked with the family again about the fact that the patient was going to die soon and there was little they could do other than increase his pain medication. The wife agreed.

"Yes, the discussion had been had. But, in that moment when you're looking at someone you love and they're cold, blue and not breathing properly, you can feel that life force seeping out of the room. You can't just sit there and watch that without doing something. It's almost against human nature to be completely calm and accepting in that moment."

This, Kaplan says, is the moment when an advance directive might not be followed. Often it's because the family won't or can't accept that their loved one is dying—or in some cases, hasn't been told that death is imminent.

COMMUNICATION RULES

In another situation, Kaplan had a patient who also had requested a DNR and was

TIPS/TOOLBOX

DISCUSSION STRATEGIES

1 **Ask patients if they have written down** their instructions when they say they have discussed advance directives with their families. Ask if the instructions continue to reflect their wishes today.

2 **Document when discussions** about advance directives have occurred. Be sure to let everyone involved, such as loved ones, spiritual leaders and the healthcare team, know.

3 **Be prepared to deal** with family members who may not want to let go of their loved one.

4 **Speak with candor** and compassion about the reality of the situation. Don't take personally words that are spoken in anger.

5 **Don't second-guess yourself—** there are no right or wrong answers, and whatever decision is made is the right decision at that time.

6 **Something can always** be done to support dying patients, such as pain medication for the patient or consolation for the family. This is an opportunity for patient and family advocacy.

RESOURCES

To access a fact sheet on advance directives, visit the National Cancer Institute at
cancer.gov/cancertopics/factsheet/Support/advance-directives.

The American Cancer Society provides information on advance care planning at
**cancer.org/Treatment/FindingandPayingforTreatment/
UnderstandingFinancialandLegalMatters/AdvanceDirectives/index**.

For more information on advance directives, see the American Society of Clinical Oncology at
cancer.net/patient/Coping/End-of-Life+Care/Advance+Directives.

The National Hospice and Palliative Care Organization has a brochure on end-of-life decisions at
caringinfo.org/files/public/brochures/End-of-Life_Decisions.pdf.

CURE ARTICLES

"Speak for Yourself" BY LAURA BEIL, 2011
curetoday.com/index.cfm/fuseaction/article.show/id/2/article_id/1725

"Speaking Out: Do's and Don'ts" BY RONALD CROSSNO, MD, CMD, 2011
curetoday.com/index.cfm/fuseaction/article.show/id/2/article_id/1701

"Q & A: Medicare and Advance Care Planning" BY LEN LICHTENFELD, MD, 2011
curetoday.com/index.cfm/fuseaction/article.show/id/2/article_id/1657

not doing well. His estranged son had come to visit him, and they were in the process of reconciling when the patient began dying. "The son looked at me and said, 'Do something,' just like that. The advance directive was not in writing. The physician came and said to him, 'You know, I had this discussion with your father, and he did not want to be on a breathing machine.' And after five minutes, the son was like, 'Okay, I understand.'"

Communication, Kaplan says, trumps documentation. Because the man had discussed his intentions with his physician and because the physician knew clearly what he wanted, he was able to speak with authority. Without it, Kaplan says, she would have had to respond to the son's wishes.

"The point is not the piece of paper; the point is the discussion. And once you've had that discussion, it needs to be documented in the progress notes. Make sure you pass that conversation on to the physician, social worker and everybody else," says Kaplan,

---

Doctors, like nurses, come with varying abilities to face death, and for some, talking about dying is very difficult.

---

noting that the document should be clearly visible in the chart.

Kaplan points out that nurses still face this challenge even when advance directives are written out because of the uncertainty of exactly when such orders should be put into place. This is when the nurses become the patient's advocate, which sometimes means telling the family their loved one is dying.

Kaplan says doctors, like nurses, come with varying abilities to face death, and for some, talking about dying is very difficult.

"Doctors are trained to make people better. I made rounds with one doctor who was visiting with a man who was clearly dying. His wife tells me the doctor said he was going to get better, the chemotherapy was going to work," Kaplan says.

"I literally had to take this woman out of the room and explain that when he stopped

48

breathing, if she kept him at full code, the team was going to come in and compress his chest bone, his sternum, and he might bleed into his heart and die that way. She was upset, and said, 'Oh, I didn't realize that.'"

ADVOCATING FOR PATIENTS

Ironically, Kaplan says, the nurse may also need to be the patient's advocate in not applying advance directives. She recounts the story of a prostate cancer patient who had come to the hospital to die after three years of hospice care. He had declined treatment earlier and told his healthcare team he just wanted to be kept comfortable. The doctor had ordered a morphine drip, which surprised Kaplan because the patient was completely awake, alert and coherent.

"I'm doing the admission assessment. I'm getting his whole history. Then I said to him, 'Well, did anybody ever offer you any treatment?' And he said, 'They talked about chemotherapy, but they said I'd be sick. Then they said radiation and said I'd be sick. I really didn't want to be sick.' I said, 'Well, haven't you been sick this whole time?' He goes, 'Yeah, kind of.'" In talking further, Kaplan learned the man's daughter was expecting her first child, and he wanted to see the baby.

"I said, 'There could be some treatment available, and maybe you could live to see that.' And he said, 'Really?' 'Yeah, really.' I spoke to the oncologist, and I said, 'Listen, you know, he's not quite ready yet.'"

The oncologist began drug therapy and rescinded the morphine drip. The man lived another 18 months. Then the family had a hard time letting him go because, in their eyes, they had had a miracle, and they wanted another one. At that point, Kaplan reminded them that, according to the man's advance directive, he did not want to suffer or be dependent on any sort of machinery.

This is only one example of how complicated such decisions can become, she says. She encourages nurses to become adept at providing therapeutic communication when confirming a patient's end-of-life wishes: "No matter how much conversation you're having with someone, if they're not listening, it really doesn't matter. So, it's the nurse [who must be] the point person at the bedside taking care of that person." ☜

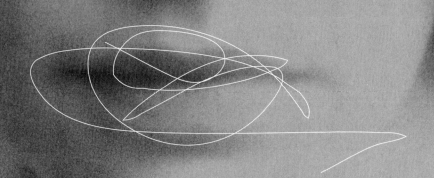

[*Chapter 7*]

On Death
and Dying

[*Chapter 7*]

On Death and Dying

O f all the difficult conversations nurses have with patients, talking about dying might be the toughest, but it is also the most important when facing advancing disease, says Tani Bahti, a registered nurse who is certified in thanatology, the study of death and dying, and in hospice and palliative care nursing.

Bahti says it is also a conversation too easily avoided. Dying is a natural part of the life cycle and should be talked about so that it can be prepared for with the same respectful attention, knowledge and caring as other significant rites of passage.

Since each person brings his or her unique history, issues, family dynamics, beliefs and traditions to life, each of these must be understood and respected as death approaches. Bahti recognizes that it's difficult for nurses to discuss dying with their patients but says that by avoiding the subject, nurses lose the opportunity to help patients make decisions and clarify their goals to find closure at the end of life.

"This conversation is critical if we are to seek a collaborative partnership that honors each person's traditions, values and goals and respects autonomy and promotes truly informed choices," she says.

DISCUSSING DEATH

When it comes to the discussion of dying, Bahti offers nurses some practical recommendations to help connect with patients. "To have the conversation about dying, you have to sit down and be eye level with the patient," Bahti says. "It gives the message that there is time, and you care enough to listen."

Bahti then asks about their illness, "Tell me what you've been told about your disease."

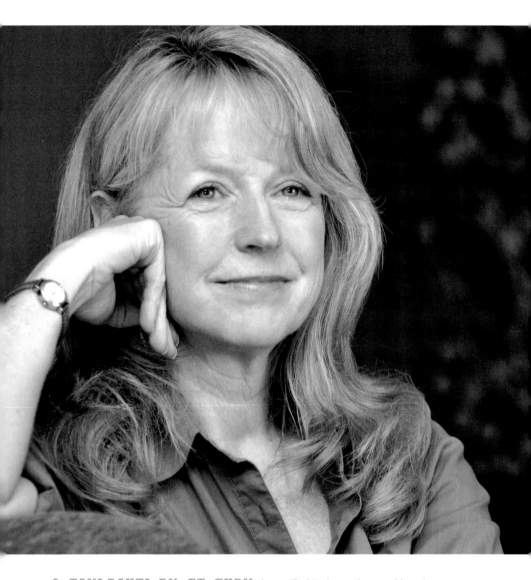

TANI BAHTI, RN, CT, CHPN, is certified in thanatology and hospice and palliative nursing. She has promoted professional and lay education on death and dying for most of her 36 years in nursing and produced the Straight Talk Series on End of Life Issues. Bahti is also founder and executive director of Passages, a nonprofit organization with a mission to provide compassionate guidance in end-of-life issues through support, education and research.

Followed by, "Tell me what you've been told about the treatment or what to expect—what is the goal?" By listening, the nurse can determine the patient's understanding and any information gaps.

"I may say, 'When I look at your records, it seems like you've been through a lot lately. What has this been like for you?' It acknowledges that they are dealing with a lot, and I want to know more about it," Bahti says. She then asks patients what they are hoping for—cure, time or just comfort with improved symptom management. After they respond, she asks, "What if it doesn't work? What are your biggest concerns or fears?"

At this point, she says, let them talk, and then ask how you can be of assistance resolving their concerns. This may require the nurse to turn to local community resources since a patient's concern or fear often has to do with issues, such as caring for dependent family members. In situations such as these, she says, patients may say they need to keep having treatment so they can stay alive for the sake of their loved ones. Informing them about available options and support may relieve some of the pressure.

Although talking about death can be difficult, not talking about it can be worse, Bahti says. "On a Saturday, we got a call from a man, and he says, 'Can somebody please check my wife? I'm not sure she's breathing.' She was not in hospice. They were from the community and didn't know where to go or what to do. I got there, and this woman was dying."

When Bahti arrived at their home, the woman was jaundiced, which led Bahti to believe that her cancer had metastasized to her liver. She was fighting to remain conscious, and her husband was still trying to get her to eat, despite her weak refusals. He explained that he was taking her to a different cancer center on Monday, and the doctors had said to keep up her strength and make sure she ate regularly. He was desperate and scared.

Bahti says that in this case, she didn't have the luxury of time to explore all the issues but needed to take quick action. "I had to say, 'It isn't going to happen.' I had to be very direct because we needed to move quickly. I told her husband, 'Her body is shutting down. She's dying. Let's talk about what we can do for comfort.' I had to explain that when the body is shutting down, food is not a benefit that will provide strength. In fact,

TIPS/TOOLBOX

DISCUSSION STRATEGIES

1 **Learn about and respect** the dying process.

2 **Sit down and talk** to patients at eye level.

3 **Ask patients where they are,** what they understand and hope for—and they will tell you.

4 **Don't be afraid to talk** about dying.

RESOURCES

The National Cancer Institute provides information on the "Last Days of Life" for patients and healthcare professionals at
cancer.gov/cancertopics/pdq/supportivecare/lasthours/patient.

The American Cancer Society's "Nearing the End of Life" gives information on what to expect in the final months of life and how to cope with death at
cancer.org/Treatment/NearingtheEndofLife/index.

The National Institute on Aging offers signs that death is approaching at
www.nia.nih.gov/HealthInformation/Publications/endoflife/05_what.htm.

For more information and resources on end-of-life issues, visit Medline Plus at
nlm.nih.gov/medlineplus/endoflifeissues.html.

CURE ARTICLES

"The Final Journey" BY KATHY LaTOUR, 2009
curetoday.com/index.cfm/fuseaction/article.show/id/2/article_id/980

"Confronting Death" BY JO CAVALLO, 2006
curetoday.com/index.cfm/fuseaction/article.show/id/2/article id/224

"A Different Kind of Caring" BY LAURA BEIL, 2006
curetoday.com/index.cfm/fuseaction/article.show/id/2/article_id/255

"Grief Before Death" BY MARC SILVER, 2007
curetoday.com/index.cfm/fuseaction/journey.showArticle/id/9/enableStageSubMenu/7/article_id/208

"Deconstructing Grief" BY ERIK NESS, 2009
curetoday.com/index.cfm/fuseaction/article.show/id/2/article_id/1248

it may increase discomfort and even tumor growth."

Bahti says the husband was distraught because he knew instinctively that she was dying. Bahti began the process of admitting her to hospice home care. "We worked quickly to get the equipment and needed medications out there. She died just 26 hours later, in the hospital bed in the living room, surrounded by family and enfolded comfortably and lovingly in the arms of her husband. It was a good ending, but he kept saying, 'Why didn't anybody tell me she was dying? Why didn't anyone tell me that forcing food would make her feel bad? If I had only known, I wouldn't have done it. I thought I was doing the right thing. Why didn't anybody tell me? Why wasn't I prepared?'"

BEING PREPARED

Bahti says she does not avoid the word death but first uses language that the patient is comfortable hearing. She has learned that when she asks questions like, "What are the changes that you are experiencing?" or "What do you think is happening?" that very often the patient will say, "I think I'm not doing well," or "I think I'm dying." She says, "Then we can follow that opening: 'If you are dying, what are your biggest fears or needs?'"

"I can remember a 74-year-old man in the hospital with widely metastatic cancer in addition to his heart and lung diseases. I'd worked with the family for about ten days back and forth about hospice. On the last day I visited, the patient was gasping for air, minimally conscious and you could feel his spirit leaving. I told the family directly that he was dying and asked what they wanted to do. The wife and daughter knew in their guts he was dying. They wanted the best care. They wanted to honor his wishes. They didn't want to do any more treatment that made him more uncomfortable, but the oncologist kept saying he could do more, that the patient 'still had time.' Despite their own deep knowing, the words of the oncologist kept them from transferring him to the hospice inpatient unit where emotional and physical care would have been available. The patient died two hours later."

The family was angry and resentful, Bahti says. "Sometimes despite the best advocating, what we may deem as 'bad deaths' happen. We must then focus on the survivors and support them, while being careful to not create more guilt and pain. I may say, 'You clearly loved [this person] and hoped for the best care and outcome. I know you got conflicting information, but you made the best decision that you possibly could on what you were told.'"

WHEN DOES TREATMENT END?

In advanced cancer, Bahti says, nurses must help people weigh the benefit and burden of treatment and to know their options. To do this takes understanding their goals. If they want to go on a family trip or attend a wedding, will the proposed treatment help them achieve that goal comfortably and safely?

"There's a point at which we need to stop doing to them if we're not actually doing for them. It's not my decision or values that count, but those of the patient, and I need to make sure they are truly informed and also prepared for any outcome."

It is important to understand the family dynamics, Bahti says. "Mom may say, 'I don't want anymore. I don't need anymore. I feel awful, but oh, my poor kids are not ready to let me go.' And sometimes moms will suffer forever until the children are ready to let them go."

Meanwhile, the children may be saying, "Mom, Dad died last year. You're all we have left. You need to live." A nurse might say, "I can see how much you love your mom, and this has to be very hard to think about losing her. Tell me about what she did best as your mother." Storytelling helps them process their grief, which must be diffused before moving to the next step: "I can hear how much you love your mother. No doubt she deserves the best possible care. Since that is what we all want, let's talk about what that care may look like."

"You can prepare them and then reinforce a decision to let go with constant affirmation: 'This has got to be difficult, but you're doing a great job. You're really honoring or keeping your loved one comfortable.' Families need to keep hearing it, that they're doing what's right because they are so scared that they've made a wrong decision, that they've stopped treatment too soon. They need a lot of supportive reinforcement."

When the patient and family know the reality, the nurse can address the fears or goals that will lead to a resolved death. According to a study published in the *Journal of the American Medical Association*, end-of-life discussions mean less use of futile treatment, which is associated with an earlier admittance into hospice and better quality of life. Another study, published in the *Journal of Pain and Symptom Management*, found that terminally ill patients who received hospice services lived on average 29 days longer than those who did not.

Hospice also allows education about the end of life, Bahti says and adds that dying from cancer is a gradual process, unlike a sudden heart attack. Families want to know what will happen but are often afraid to ask. "Hospice benefits all around. It doesn't take away hope. It gives them a choice and respect and time for closure."

Bahti recalls a young mother who was able to say, "I'm not going to be here when my kids grow up." This allowed her to focus on deciding how she would leave her legacy: the pictures and the letters she wanted to prepare for their birthdays, weddings and more.

"She really got involved with making sure that she lived for her children, and that was a wonderful example of closure I then shared with other patients: What's the message they want to leave? Where do they want to die? And if it's a young person, what about their kids? Or it may be an older person who asks, 'what about my dog or cat?'"

Bahti says these issues can affect the advance directive, with people changing their minds in both directions. "That's why hospice should go into the preparation because it's usually when they're scared or there's been a drama that they panic and say, 'Oh my God. Not yet. Not now.' It's nice to have somebody that says, 'Remember we talked about the changes.'"

It may never be "okay" to let a loved one die but allowing for that release into death may be important. Bahti talks of a woman who was dying at age 46. "Her 20-year-old daughter had lymphoma, and she had an 18-year-old son. Both knew their mom was dying, but just the same, they would go into her room and say, 'You're going to be okay, Mom. We'll get you stronger.'"

Bahti pulled the husband aside and explained what she had heard. He talked to the children and they went back in and very tearfully said, 'We love you, Mom and, we are really going to miss you, but we'll be okay.' The woman visibly relaxed and died ten minutes later.

"To die, people need to let go on three levels," Bahti says. "First, you need to let go of grandma. Then, grandma needs to let go of you. Finally, grandma's body needs to let go of her. So I encourage families who I see holding on, to find their own way of releasing and to know that each person has their own timing to letting go."

THE PROCESS OF DYING

The discussion about the physical act of dying comes early for Bahti, often on the first visit to a patient in hospice care, because it eases the patient's mind about what to expect. "I'll usually say, 'You know, I understand that there's a lot of concerns and questions about the process of dying. Would you like to know what to expect?' And then I get that little imperceptible nod that says, 'I didn't know I was allowed to ask.'"

Bahti goes through how the disease will progress, what changes to expect and how they will be managed—and then what dying will be like.

"I talk about paying attention to the body and not intervening, but maintaining comfort," Bahti says. "And I talk about the fact that ultimately just about everybody goes into that wonderful coma before they die." Bahti speaks of the wonders of the body and how it cares for patients as they die. She talks about death as going to sleep, whether it is for minutes or days, while the body shuts down. "Then the patient can breathe easier, and the family is okay, since they know the patient won't drop dead at the dinner table. They begin sensing that they can do this."

For nurses, the most important thing is honoring the body's wisdom and knowing that they can keep them comfortable, Bahti says. "And if the patient is in hospice, we'll be with them every step of the way."

Nurses are often told that they need to be emotionally detached from the dying process, but Bahti says nurses who do not connect can't have that level of conversation where healing occurs. She describes her personal philosophy as "if you do not wear your heart on your sleeve, you don't belong in health care. We must be healers, and that can only happen through heartfelt connection, human being to human being." ∽

Notes

At Genentech BioOncology™, we're leading the fight against cancer with innovative science and fundamentally transforming the way cancer is treated. Our commitment to this goal has enabled us to make significant contributions to the understanding of cancer and to translate this understanding into targeted, biologic-based therapies.

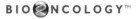

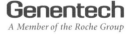